Wounded Nostalgia

Eugenio Borgna
Translated by Jamie Richards
and Adrian Nathan West

Wounded Nostalgia

La nostalgia ferita

PETER LANG

Bruxelles · Berlin · Chennai · Lausanne · New York · Oxford

Bibliographic information published by the Deutsche Nationalbibliothek.
The German National Library lists this publication in the German National Bibliography;
detailed bibliographic data is available on the Internet at http://dnb.d-nb.de.

Library of Congress Cataloging-in-Publication Data
LCCN: 2025049024

This book has been translated thanks to a grant from the Italian Ministry of Foreign Affairs
and International Cooperation.

La nostalgia ferita
© 2018 Giulio Einaudi editore s.p.a., Torino

ISBN 978-3-0343-5104-1 (Print)
ISBN 978-3-0343-5105-8 (ePDF)
ISBN 978-3-0343-5106-5 (ePub)
DOI 10.3726/b23362
Dépôt légal D/2025/5678/66

© 2026 Peter Lang Group AG, Lausanne, (Switzerland)
Published by P.I.E. PETER LANG s.a., Brussels (Belgium)

info@peterlang.com

www.peterlang.com

Contents

Preface

Michele Dantini

Of Eugenio Borgna, we appreciate his objectivity and composure, the *measure* that gives his texts, never caustic or brutal, the hushed tone of quiet reflection. Yet this moderation conceals a great radicalism. If there is such a thing as an intimately relational psychiatry, based on listening, "humanistic" and anti-authoritarian, this is precisely the psychiatry to associate with Borgna. He invites the psychiatrist to lay down the usual shields of the profession— jargon, statistics, diagnostic tools—and contend first and foremost with the patient's suffering, acknowledging it not as something alien, but possible, human, of one's own. The therapeutic relationship thus becomes authentically existential: a process of "healing" and discovery in which the psychiatrist, having excluded any presumptions of foreknowledge or certainty, takes part, in an almost Socratic way, through a shared process of recollection.

Humanity itself, understood in terms of "finitude," "thrownness," "angst," or other analytical-existential categories we could trace back (as does Borgna) to early twentieth-century philosophy, is revealed as a common *wound*, the origin that makes relationality and listening itself, both in everyday and clinical terms, possible. Borgna conserves from these philosophers of existence—Heidegger, but also Jaspers and others—the specifically psychological and moral core, and from the Italian tradition (particularly from Turin and Luigi Pareyson) of "positive existentialism," draws his anti-dogmatic stance and clinical model—put simply, solidarity put into practice.

Relevant here is the passion with which Borgna, in his introduction to my book *Sulla delicatezza* [On Delicacy] (Il Mulino 2021), responds to my discussion of Socrates and Dostoevsky, particularly on the *agape* (or "benevolence," in Borgna's terms) that Myshkin and then Alyosha Karamazov show those they encounter who are distrustful, contrarian, or hostile: proof not so much of Borgna's extensive philosophical and literary background, so evident to readers it doesn't bear mention, but of the importance that certain "classics" of Western culture have had in his formation, an importance equal (or perhaps greater) to that of the specialist literature of the field. Something like an inexorable *esprit de finesse*, in Borgna's eyes, reigns supreme, above and beyond any "discourse on [psychiatric] method."

Following this, one may, or perhaps must, question Borgna's "ideology," fundamental to understanding his more political psychiatric interventions, particularly his initial support and subsequent reservations about the Basaglia law, or its implementation, which, notwithstanding the merits of the original proposal, due to a lack of public resources allocated ad hoc or otherwise, failed to serve patients in the difficult process of post-asylum social reintegration. Borgna's attitude is commendably anti-doctrinal, and the reasons for his "militant" point of view are supported concretely by the everyday circumstances of patients and families.

Borgna merges moderation and radicalism in unusual ways, in no way pandering to popular opinion, but on the contrary, by rejecting or emending the buzzwords and commonplaces of academia and the media.

A Nostalgia That Never Dies

Looking back at my adolescence, immersing myself in the depths of the past, I cannot but recall the impact of the September 8, 1943 armistice and the Resistance thereafter. My father had to leave our city and home, because the Germans, who knew his political position, were in pursuit of him; I was only thirteen, my youngest brother wasn't even two, but we, my siblings and mother and I, were forced to abandon our house with its big garden, its ancient trees, and take refuge in a small town tucked into a green hill from which Lake Orta and San Giulio Island, with its dreamlike, mystic grace, were visible in the distance, with the glow of the Benedictine monastery that made it seem even more arcane. The green of the hill, strikingly luminous, became brighter by the light of spring, and the silence, austere and lingering, surrounded us, and it seemed as if we were in another world. Nothing broke that silence but birdsong and greetings called out by the few hands working in the fields. There were no more German soldiers, no more checkpoints, no more mounting fear and anguish such as was spreading in the city where we'd lived before. With the help of her sister, eleven years older, and of friends who ignored danger to visit us, my mother managed to arrange a life for us, and to allow us to read and study in the months of our exile. On the surface, nothing in our family life had changed, and yet we were tormented by my father's absence; my father, from the mountains in Ossola, where he had joined up with other Catholic partisans, had no way to communicate anything about his life to us. And then there was the anxiety of the Germans' sudden raids on our enchanted village and the house where we were staying. I cannot forget how slowly the days passed, and the sound of bells, almost like the blue bells of Trakl, from a church nearby, or actually next door, accompanying our nights, sometimes keeping us up; and how the endless clear and bright mornings, in that silent spring, followed one after the other, sending subdued, harmonious echoes down the valley that descended almost to the edge of the lake and died in its never-agitated waters, which were always meek and mute. The mornings were ours, and our endless walks transported us along mysterious forest paths where the chanting of birds surrounded us. In the afternoons, we read and studied, and we listened to the radio: the news, which Swiss radio carried, and which we heard with bated breath. That was my life, our life, in those long months of exile, which still burn brightly in my memory, uninterrupted by gaps of forgetting. My adolescence was shaped by this period of my life that confronted me with changes in the experience of time, not clock-time but inner time, which passed slowly in town, slower than in our city, a time described by Thomas Mann in his most fascinating novel, *The Magic Mountain*, in which I sometimes saw myself. As a teenager, I was already reading books, poetry, novels, essays, which my father would bring home from his frequent visits to the bookstore, and some of these books accompanied us in our exile. Then, one day, one happy day, peace came, my father returned from the mountains, and we reunited in our abandoned home, which the Germans had ravaged, using it as a military post. Life began again, school began again, the church bells were no longer blue and strident, the nights passed in silence, we played tennis again, and the hours, light and dark, began to reel past again in the wake of a time that opened up ever more toward the future, but was shaded, gradually, by the colors of a past consumed by nostalgia. Yes, the waves of life are unpredictable, as in the beautiful, immortal novel by Virginia Woolf, and nostalgia for those months of exile has never vanished from my memory, however true it is that when I was there, in that little town, what I longed for was our big house with the immense garden and the tennis court, and the lindens, the walnuts and chestnuts and firs, which even today rise up in the sky, ethereal; and then there was the room where I studied, from which I could glimpse Monte Rosa blanketed in perennial snow, on sunny days in summer and winter, capturing the final rays that shot across the sky. Of course, one longs for that age burnt by the years, for the ashes of adolescence, and yet it is those experiences, remote in time, that give us the occasion to reflect on the meaning of life and death, hope and despair, isolation and solitude. A living nostalgia, one that never dies in us? Perhaps.

On the Threshold

Nostalgia is a vital state none of us can elude in the infinite unfurling of life. Nostalgia, and in particular nostalgia wounded by the passage of time, which amplifies it, makes it increasingly bitter and painful, fragile and arcane, is woven through with memories of the past unrelated to the future: a past bright and shimmering or else dark and painful, born and dying like fragile and ephemeral butterflies, ethereal and ungraspable. Nostalgia is a key term made up of myriad interwoven semantic sources, which I will set out to analyze and describe following a mysterious path that leads into the core of existence: interiority. And yet to speak of interiority means taking the hard, painful road of self-awareness, questioning the modes of this awareness and its relationship to the awareness of others, confronting the emotions and passions that are inside ourselves and everyone else.

Emotional Awareness

To rational awareness, and not only in psychology, we must add emotional awareness, the awareness that is drawn along by the emotions and the passions, as Giacomo Leopardi says, and as we find in *The Confusions of Young Törless*, one of the most fascinating works by Robert Musil, author of the incomparable modern literary classic *The Man Without Qualities*. I would like to excerpt here an extraordinary passage that examines the problem of rational and emotional awareness: "For it is strange how it is with thoughts. They are often no more than accidentals that fade out again without leaving any trace; and thoughts have their dead and their vital seasons. We sometimes have a flash of understanding that amounts to the insight of genius, and yet it slowly withers, even in our hands—like a flower. The form remains, but the colors and the fragrance are gone. That is to say, we still remember it all, word for word, and the logical value of the proposition, the discovery, remains entirely unimpaired, and nevertheless it merely drifts aimlessly about on the surface of our mind, and we do not feel ourselves any the richer for it. And then, perhaps years later—all at once there is again a moment when we see that in the meantime we have known nothing of it, although in terms of logic we have known it all."

Musil continues powerfully: "Yes, there are dead and living thoughts. The process of thinking that takes place on the illumined surface, and which can always be checked and tested by means of the thread of causality, is not necessarily the living one. A thought that one encounters in this way remains as much a matter of indifference as any given man in a column of marching soldiers. Although a thought may have entered our brain a long time earlier, it comes to life only in the moment when something that is no longer thought, something that is not merely logical, combines with it and makes us feel its truth beyond the realm of all justification, as though it had dropped an anchor that tore into the blood-warm, living flesh...."

He concludes: "Any great flash of understanding is only half completed in the illumined circle of the conscious mind; the other half takes place in the dark loam of our innermost being. It is primarily a state of soul, and uppermost, as it were at the extreme tip of it, there the thought is poised like a flower."

Historical Outlines

Nostalgia (from the Greek *nostos*, return, and *algos*, pain) is a complex emotion with multiple resonances in which conflicting ways of being and living converge. The word appears for the first time in 1688 in a medical dissertation defended at the University of Basel by Johannes Hofer, who treats it as an illness, and he chooses this name for it to emphasize the pain caused by distance and the burning desire of *Heimweh*, the yearning for home. The story is reconstructed along with an archeology of nostalgia in a book by Jean Starobinski with beautiful pages on the history and phenomenology of melancholy. Before becoming the word that, today, denotes a sphere of great, ineffable emotional significance, nostalgia was deemed an illness in the medical literature. Obviously, this definition faded over the course of time. But Starobinski maintains that even before this medical characterization, nostalgia had a more general name in Latin, namely desire, which even today is not irrelevant to the multiple semantic connotations of nostalgia.

Images of Nostalgia

There is not one single nostalgia: it comes, instead, in infinite forms, and is an experience that it is impossible not to come across in certain moments, in certain seasons of our lives; and is it not the passion of phenomenology, as Moritz Geiger has written, to describe and, for that matter, discern the differences between them? There is the nostalgia for childhood once lived, which lives in us, arcane and secret in memory. There is the nostalgia for the beloved, distant or deceased, who is no longer with us; there is the nostalgia for a former home, full of memories that still accompany us on our path with their lights and shadows, with their swarms of emotions lost and searched for again in vain; and there is a still more painful nostalgia: the one that leads to illness and depression, that is itself an illness of body and soul. There is the nostalgia for music, for landscapes, for enchanted mountains still visible in their immobile remoteness though they can no longer be reached, nostalgia for the high tides that have washed over our perspectives and bathed us in the silence and stupor of the heart. There is a nostalgia for the places that witnessed the flourishing of our adolescence and youth and hopes, places that are gone but live on, luminous and intact, in the occasionally wounded memory of fate. There is a nostalgia of experiences that nurtured our souls, experiences that have faded to embers that never die out and may unexpectedly flare up again. There is nostalgia for the lost homeland, where we were born, where we've lived, places we've left or have been forced to leave, as happens more and more nowadays in distant lands devastated by violence and death.

Beyond their various existential roots, there are forms of nostalgia like endless archipelagos that help us live, that compel us to look at the past, to draw images from it, and give us meaning, by helping us elude the dragon of forgetting, the glaciers of lost emotions never to be found again. There are painful, gutting forms of nostalgia, and others that are dreamed or day-dreamed, nostalgias that help us to live, nostalgias that carry us into death, nostalgias nourished by glimmering recollections of joy and sorrow; nostalgias that are never erased despite the passage of time, labile and ephemeral nostalgias, Leopardian nostalgias that accompany us in every season of our lives, brightening our way with their starry glow and freeing us from the shores of emptiness where the vessels of our lives so easily flounder, where our hearts grow weary and dull.

An image, the image of the foreign soul on earth, which emerges luminously in a heart-rending poem by Georg Trakl, seems to me to lie at the roots of every form of nostalgia, in particular the longing for the homeland, the homeland of the lost heart that lives on in the memory wracked by loneliness. Spirit, transcendence, fate, alienation, distance, the yearning for return, are part of experiences enigmatically interwoven in every manner of nostalgia, and particularly in that form of it which is born painfully from the loss of one's homeland. I would like to invoke a wonderful thought of Umberto Galimberti's: "When the heart oscillates between past and present, between near and far, it is always the past, always the faraway that captures the soul, not to devour it, but to return it to its source, the auroral spring from which the new day may draw light."

Nostalgia has nothing at all to do with calculating reason; it is a matter of the ardent furnace of emotion.

The Confines of Nostalgia

In the introduction to a collection of essays about nostalgia, Rolf Petri asks himself what nostalgia is, and responds: "It is a feeling, and paradoxically this means it can only be described through words that refer to other feelings. Nostalgia is properly associated with yearning, heartache, sorrow, desire, mourning"; and, "The nostalgic feeling associated with any discourse about the past or about remoteness, however, nearly always gives rise to the hope of return or mourning for a return denied, leading not to resignation, but rather to motivation. And as every return, every recuperation, every action of salvaging, can only be realized in the future, there emerges the impossibility of dissociating the feeling of nostalgia from expectations for the future. A vigorous, utopian expectation intertwined with the idealization of places from the past, or those distant in space, that are conceived of as the bearers of memory and the portraits of desire." Yes, nostalgia is a carousel of emotions, of images, of rediscoveries, of intuitions and remembrances woven together and united, granting life to a lost or diffuse past, but without closing itself off to the future.

Now I would like to consider whether there is a difference between nostalgia and regret, or if one encroaches ceaselessly on the other. In delimiting the subject of nostalgia, I must also draw out certain fragmentary considerations on its points of consonance and dissonance with regret. Nostalgia lives on the past, as does regret, and so how can one be distinguished from the other? If dwelling in the past naturally brings together nostalgia and regret, there is, nonetheless, something that seems to separate them, as I would illustrate by turning to language, this house of being, as Martin Heidegger defines it in one of his most readily graspable texts. In nostalgia, we do not hear the echo of an acute and painful, univocal and radical emotional climax such as strikes us in regret. Our regrets pertain to a thing, a person, or a human experience that has brought meaning into our lives, in the knowledge that they are forever lost and with the sensation that we are somehow responsible for what has happened. In regret, there is a kind of mournful remembrance, a mourning for something no longer there, whereas in nostalgia, expectation abides, the hope that things lost still have meaning. In regret, we feel painfully guilty and responsible for what has been lost, and there are never the sometimes elegiac ripples of nostalgia that make us look back on our past experiences as though they continued to live on in our hearts and our memories, and that heal the wounds of the present, helping us endure the absence of people and places we have loved. Regret cannot offer us this; in regret, the past is relived in its petrified immobility, and is hardly able to exercise any influence whatsoever on the present: what we think, what we feel. These distinctions are born not of word-games, they are not fleeting and inconsistent shooting stars; rather, they help us to better understand what we are and what others are in the depths of our emotional lives. Emotions express what is occurring inside us, in our souls, but they are also forms of knowledge, and must be made to emerge from the depths of our conscious and unconscious life. Nostalgia and regret are emotions, moods, that accompany us in all stages of our lives, though we do not always seek them; yet this seeking is necessary to better understand our inner lives.

Childhood Rediscovered: The Memories That Save Us

We can get nowhere near the mysterious demarcation lines of childhood and adolescence except through the path that leads inward, to our inner selves, and I would like to reconsider this boundless subject following those experiences and modes of awareness evoked by certain texts that have accompanied me throughout my life, and continue to accompany me still. These are texts I've known since my school days, some well-known, some less so, greatly impactful on my reflections on the meaning of childhood and adolescence and the values they contain. But texts are not enough if we are to realize—*re*-think, *re*-member—the story of our childhood and adolescence. And this is not a waste of time; this is the principle by which parents and teachers, doctors and educators, know how to approach children and adolescents, particularly those who are suffering, identifying with them and trying to relive their own personal experiences from childhood and adolescence. I am talking not only of psychiatric texts, but of literary ones as well, that bring us into the mystery of childhood and adolescence.

Beautiful things about childhood, about the resonances of childhood in our lives, can be read in Fyodor Dostoevsky's moving novel, *The Brothers Karamazov*, especially in its final pages. His words, like Leopardi's, help us to retrieve something from the abysses that open before our eyes and reflect on the nostalgia for youth and its enigmatic presence in our imaginations and our lives. As when Ivan Karamazov turns to the young people who are listening to him: "My little doves—let me call you so, for you are very like them, those pretty blue birds, at this minute as I look at your good dear faces. My dear children, perhaps you won't understand what I am saying to you, because I often speak very unintelligibly, but you'll remember it all the same and will agree with my words some time." Then the image of childhood is reborn: "You must know that there is nothing higher and stronger and more wholesome and good for life in the future than some good memory, especially a memory of childhood, of home. People talk to you a great deal about your education, but some good, sacred memory, preserved from childhood, is perhaps the best education. If a man carries many such memories with him into life, he is safe to the end of his days, and if one has only one good memory left in one's heart, even that may sometime be the means of saving us." And now, Karamazov says, "Perhaps we may even grow wicked later on, may be unable to refrain from a bad action, may laugh at men's tears and at those people who say as Kolya did just now, 'I want to suffer for all men,' and may even jeer spitefully at such people. But however bad we may become—which God forbid—yet, when we recall how we buried Ilusha, how we loved him in his last days, and how we have been talking like friends all together, at this stone, the cruelest and most mocking of us—if we do become so—will not dare to laugh inwardly at having been kind and good at this moment! What's more, perhaps, that one memory may keep him from great evil and he will reflect and say, 'Yes, I was good and brave and honest then!'"

The Infinite and Memories of Childhood

I would like to excerpt from Giacomo Leopardi's *Zibaldone* certain fragments that speak of the nostalgia for childhood and youth, that age of immersion in the vague and the indefinite: "If, as children, we take delight and pleasure in a view, a landscape, a painting, a sound, etc., a story, a description, a fairy tale, a poetic image, a dream, that delight and pleasure is always vague and indefinite. The idea that is awakened in us is always indeterminate and limitless, every solace, every pleasure, every expectation, every project, illusion, etc. (indeed, almost every conception), at that age always has something of the infinite about it, and nourishes us and fills our soul in a way that cannot be put into words, even through the smallest objects. When we grow up, whether they are greater pleasures and objects, or the same ones that charmed us as children, such as a lovely view, a landscape, a painting, etc., we will feel pleasure, but it will never be comparable in any way to this sense of the infinite, or certainly it will not be so intensely, perceptibly, enduringly, and essentially vague and indeterminate."

These thoughts extend down other obscure paths that tell us how childhood memories are mirrored in the experiences and ideas that resurface in us long after childhood: "Indeed, note that possibly the majority of the indefinite images and sensations that we feel even after childhood, and throughout the rest of our life, are nothing other than a remembrance of childhood. They look back to it, depend upon and derive from it, are in a way an emanation and consequence of it, either in general or in particular. In other words, we experience that sensation, idea, pleasure, etc., because we remember, and there appears in our imagination, the same sensation, image, etc., we experienced as children, and how we experienced it in those same circumstances. So that the present sensation does not derive directly from things, it is not an image of objects, but an image of the childhood image, a recollection, a repetition, a reechoing, or reflection of the old image."

This sensation is not infrequent: "And this is a very frequent occurrence. (Thus, in my own case, if I see once more the prints that gave me such pleasure as a child, the places, sights, encounters, etc., and think back to the stories, fairy tales, books, dreams, etc., and hear again the lullabies I first heard in childhood or early youth, etc.) So that, had we not been children, we would—in our present condition—be deprived of most of those few indefinite sensations which remain to us, since we experience them only in relation to, and by virtue of, our childhood. And note that even pleasurable dreams at the age we are now, though they delight us far more than reality, nevertheless no longer represent the same indefinite beauty and pleasure that they so often had in our earliest years."

These are reflections of great depth that demonstrate once more the boundless emotional intelligence of Giacomo Leopardi, which penetrates so deeply into the most secret and shimmering meaning of interiority: his own interiority, and the interiority of others. The correlations between the oneiric world of childhood and the conscious world of adulthood are brought to life with a semantic force it is impossible to forget. Perhaps it goes without saying that the *Zibaldone*, even for a field as distant and practical as psychiatry, is an endless source of knowledge and anthropological and phenomenological reflections. Indeed, I would like to turn now to one of Leopardi's most fascinating lyrics, his "Recollections," immersed in the boundless sea of nostalgia.

Recollections

The uniting thread of Leopardi's great idylls is memory, nostalgia; this is, as it were, the germ or seed of these works, and it shines wonderfully in "The Recollections" as well. Francesco Flora's beautiful words attest to this: "'The Recollections' contains the primary essence of all Leopardian motifs. Even in terms of length, it is the poet's vastest work: it hearkens back to the very source of all poetry: childhood memory, which he always considered the native kernel of poetry. His is not a song of memories, but a song to Mnemosyne herself, the mother of poetry." And also: "He mourns youth, youth which he never had; and so, he mourns the youth he would have wanted, the youth of adolescent longing. Even the verse's material is so ethereal as to appear almost immaterial."

From this poem, I want to highlight the moments that luminously shade this nostalgia for childhood and youth, as here in the first lines of the third stanza:

> The wind comes, with the hour that tolls
> from the town tower. This sound, I can remember,
> was a comfort to my nights,
> when as a child I lay in my dark room
> prey to unrelenting terrors, sighing for morning.
> There's nothing here I see or feel
> but that some image doesn't live in me again,
> some sweet memory come to light.
> Sweet in itself; but knowledge of the present
> replaces it with pain, and a vain desire
> for the past, however sad, and the wish
> to say: I was.

The tolling of the hours comforted the poet, and in his soul, despite his unease, was reborn the sweet recollection of a luminous past: of childhood. The poet's memories are brimming with what had been the hopes of his early years, as he says at the beginning of the fourth stanza:

Hopes, hopes: O bright illusions
of my early years! Whenever I talk
I come around to you, for though time passes
and affections and ideas change,
I can't forget you. Yes, I understand
glory and honor are phantoms
joys and things mere wishes; life produces nothing,
only senseless suffering. Yet though my years
are empty, though my mortal life
is barren and lightless, I can see
that fate is taking little from me.
Yet sometimes I think back on you, old hopes of mine,
and my sweet first imagining, and then
look at my life, so purposeless, so painful,
and see that death
is what remains for me of so much hope.
I feel my heart break, and I'm totally
inconsolable about my fate.

The theme of hope is paired with that of Leopardi's youth wounded by the death of Nerina. Hopes are fragile as ever, and easily devoured by death; and the death of Nerina, her life cut short in adolescence like Silvia's, is the subject of the rending final stanza of this poem. Its emotional atmosphere grows more ardent, more suffused with nostalgia, in the moment that speaks of Nerina's incomparable grace and her cruel decline into death; but Leopardi still remembers her, feverish companion of his every vague imagining, with bitterness. This stanza is indescribably tender, and we cannot grasp its shattered beauty except in the stupefied silence of the heart.

O Nerina! Isn't it of you
I hear these places speaking?
Could I have possibly forgotten you?
Where have you gone, that all that I find here
are memories of you, my sweetness?
This Earth where you were born sees you no more:
that window where you used to talk to me,
and which reflects the sad light of the stars,
is empty. Where are you, that I no longer
hear your voice the way I did,
when the slightest murmur from your lips
would turn me pale? Another time.
Your days are over, my sweet love.

You left.
Others walk the earth today
and live in these fragrant hills.
But you went quickly; and your life
was like a dream. You danced; joy glistened
on your forehead, and that confident
imagining, the light of youth,
shone in your eyes,
till fate extinguished them
and you fell. Ah, Nerina! The old love
rules in my heart. If now and then I go
to gatherings or parties, I say to myself:
O Nerina, you no longer dress your hair
or go to gatherings. When May returns
and boys give flowering branches to their girls
and sing to them, I say: My Nerina, neither spring
nor love will ever come for you again.
Each brilliant day, each blooming hill I see,
whatever pleases me, I say:
Nothing can please Nerina now. She doesn't see
the fields, the air. You're gone,
lifelong regret of mine, you're gone;
and the bitter memory will last
with all my fond imagining, each tender feeling,
and every sad, sweet motion of my heart.

This is one of Leopardi's most fascinating poems, one we read and reread in its vertiginous alternation of themes that grade from hopes—hopes fragile and unpredictable in their birth and in death, but nonetheless impossible to eradicate (for they are part of life itself)—into painful longing for the lofty youth of Nerina struck down by death. Who can remain unmoved by the lightness and musicality of these mournful, impalpable verses that tell of life's unutterable splendor and its agonizing and fleeting brevity?

Grandmother Speranza's Friend

And how can we not hear the shaded, meek voice of nostalgia, scarlet and harmonious, echoing in the poetry of Guido Gozzano, especially in one of his most beautiful and unforgettable verses, "Grandmother Speranza's Friend"?

This poem appeared in his first collection, *The Road to Shelter*, from 1907, and was included in the second, *The Colloquies*, albeit with certain changes. Its arcane fascination, its readability, its lightness, its freshness, its weary, crepuscular climax, its song-like, haunting musicality, its almost obsessive thematic repetitions, weave together to create the miracle of a poem impregnated with nostalgia which, like the rest of his works, one feels compelled to return to as soon as one has come to know it; the same way one keeps listening to the music of Strauss under the magic, unforgettable direction of Carlos Kleiber, which brings out its vertiginous depths and its nostalgic modernity.

I would like to quote here verses from the second stanza of the poem, which are run through with the feverish nostalgia of childhood and adolescence expressed in the marvel of scintillating, phantasmagoric words—unforgettable:

The little boys have to beware when they come in the parlor
    today
(the dust covers, just for today, have been taken off all of the
    chairs).
But still they come galloping through. She's home on
    vacation (they've missed her),
Speranza is home, their big sister! Her comrade Carlotta's
    here too!
My Grandmother's seventeen now. Carlotta is almost as old:
    and not long ago they were told that hoop skirts would now
    be allowed.
Now the widest of hoops ripples under a skirt lined with
    Cobalt blue roses,
while crinoline tightly encloses a wasp-waist incredibly
    slender.
They've shawls decorated with little flowers oranges birds
    everywhere,
and they wear all the way to the middle of their cheeks the
    two bands of their hair.
Their exams were the finest of all in their class. What a
    terrible few
days they have just suffered through! Now they're finished
    forever with school.
Now children, be still if you please! The two—now be quiet,
    I say!—
the two friends are going to play some songs from the long-
    ago days.

And in closing:

> Carlotta sings, while Speranza plays piano. And in the brief
>   song
> flowering life opens its hands as its thousand bright promises
>   throng.
> In the music's susurrus they see, each one in her soul's secret
>   place,
> a smile just for her on the face of Prince Charming, her
>   husband-to-be,
> the husband who's kissed her already, in dreams . . . In the
>   long days at school
> all the petals of daisies they pulled to the tenderest verses of
>   Prati!

The fifth and final stanza is marked by a nostalgia that, as through a glass darkly, is the image and metaphor of spiritual pain and everyday suffering; and are these not the leitmotifs of Guido Gozzano's inspired lyrics?

> Carlotta! Your name's not a song, but like a rare perfume it
>   calls
> up a world of young women in shawls and diligences
>   creaking along . . .
> Friend of Grandmother Speranza, I walk past the flower beds
>   where
> you read of young Ortis' despair in Foscolo's tender romance.
>   Here you are in the album: it gives me such sadness to look at
> the date written there in your hand: *twenty-eighth of June eighteen
>   hundred and fifty.*
> As if rapt in a lyric, impassioned, you gaze heavenward, with
>   one small
> finger beside your lips, all in the height of a long-ago fashion.
> That day—melancholy reflections possess me now—you were
>   arrayed
> all in pink for the portrait they made with the *camera*—the
>   latest invention.
> But 1 can't find you now in your prime, Grandmother's
>   friend! Where've you gone,
> you who might be the woman, the one I could love, I could
>   love for all time?

A bitter, fluid nostalgia abounds in this poem, interspersed with extenu-
ated and intermittent sorrow, at once luminous and frayed, bordering the
impossibility of love.

Oh, Hours of Childhood

In this context, how can we not think of the hours of solitude that form
part of our lives, and of that warm companionship we receive from thinking
about the past, that gentle, ineffable nostalgia that fills them and helps us to
feel less alone? Nostalgia, unlike regret, is a product of lived experience and
unrealized but lingering hopes, of images and places, faces and tears, smiles
and gestures that have filled the seasons of our lives, above all from our
childhood and youth, which continue to live in memory and in the eyes of
the soul and sometimes seem to us to persist in reality. When the dark night
of the soul descends upon us, if we cannot draw on the grace and shadows of
nostalgia, of the recapture of a distant, shimmering past, how can we place
hope in a future that will give meaning to our lives? How can we not speak
of nostalgia for the sea, the silent sea with its infinitude that mysteriously
reopens our hearts to hopes neglected, perhaps impossible, but that help us
to live, or at least survive? When we feel nostalgia for places, the sea, people
or emotions from the distant past, does it not become like seeing them again,
and in the light that they emanate? Thinking back to that period after the
war, those of bright and ineffable months of vacation when we were carefree
at our house in Liguria on a bluff overlooking the stark sea rocks in their
eternal silence, I cannot but feel nostalgia, a nostalgia that is painful and yet
generative, salvaging the past and restoring it to its restless fluctuations and
broken hopes. In short, there is the nostalgia that hurts, the nostalgia that
sometimes becomes an illness, but there is also the nostalgia that urges us
to live, and revives within us a past that would otherwise be lost forever. In
the wake of memory and the nostalgia that breathes scintillating life into it,
I see myself again on those same seaside rocks, reading for hours, immersed
in the silence of the heart, lulled by the crashing of the waves, reading novels
and stories and especially poetry, which the sea helped me to take in, with
its transparency and musicality. Such heights of emotion I was only able to
experience in those hours, on those days, with their unforgettable charm

and magic, that the murky waves of nostalgia allowed me—and sometimes still do—to relive, to revive from the silence and oblivion that so hungrily and cruelly devour even the most luminous past.

In the fourth of Rainer Maria Rilke's *Duino Elegies*, there is a fragile, arcane image of the nostalgia for childhood that rouses indescribable emotions:

> O hours of childhood, when more than the mere past was behind
> each shape and the future wasn't stretched out
> before us. We were growing; sometimes we hurried
> to grow up too soon, half for the sake of those
> who had nothing more than being grown-up. Yet when we were alone, we still amused
> ourselves with the everlasting and stood there
> in that gap between world and toy,
> in a place which, from the very start,
> had been established for a pure event.

Rilke's nostalgia for childhood, the nostalgia for childhood and youth in Proust—with their haunting allure and infinite hopes that naturally always risk turning to bright illusions—are not so easily struck from our memory or our lives, and Rilke's words repeat all this with their shrill timbre, at times unfathomable in its mystery.

Like a Shooting Star

Desires, expectations, draw nourishment not only from the future, but also from the past, from things that have been as much as from things that are yet to be. Nostalgia suffuses the liquid and fragile fabric of desire, desire for things we've lost and that we'd like to have again. There is no nostalgia that is not fed by the past, the Augustinian present of the past, and that does not believe it cannot be revived; indeed, sometimes it is. It strikes me that perhaps Rilke's beautiful novel *The Notebooks of Malte Laurids Brigge*, which I have continued to read since my schooldays, is submerged in the Heraclitean river of generative nostalgia that brings back to life the past, the emotions and the moods that were linked to the past and that fill our inner lives, stretching their boundaries and reinvigorating them with new blood.

What do the thematic declinations of this devastating and at times unfathomable novel tell us? That in life we are alone, for one, and no one notices us, our anxieties or our pains, our all-consuming nostalgia; but also that no one notices the stars that fall in silence on the night of San Lorenzo; that no one remembers to make a wish. Rilke's ardent, broken words are ones we cannot easily forget, and we must keep them burning in our hearts and minds, because in them, in the inexpressible glow of the images they evoke, we see the delicate trace of nostalgia with its chameleonic emotional resonances and its airy fragility. Nostalgia for the past, for the past of adolescence, emerges painfully from these pages that show us how prose can become poetry, poetry shimmering with metaphor, transformed by language of oneiric immediacy and high lyrical tension. Rilke's novel is ultimately a meta-novel, unfolding in fragile words and phosphorescent images animated by a fervent nostalgia of gentleness and compassion, lightness, and liquidity: in other words, grace.

What does the great writer Claudio Magris have to say about this extraordinary novel? "The existence of Malte, prototype of the modern subject with no home and no identity, is one of estrangement, the loss of a childhood and an individuality that he never actually possessed other than through nostalgia. Malta lives in nostalgia for a life which is always elsewhere. He seeks the meaning of his existence in memories or the objects of others, in family recollections, in historical traditions; even his own life is in its entirety a simple 'mute and nameless' lament for life, as in Hofmannsthal's poem." And later: "Malte's nostalgia is directed toward an existence that has never been, a fulfillment that was awaited and mourned without ever arriving. Living, for Malte, means distancing himself from life, constantly taking leave of it. 'When is the present?' Rilke wonders, a bit like when Oblomov asks himself: 'When does one live?' For Malte, the only present is that of words, which he writes remembering or imagining life—that is, the present of writing. Life is only remembered in itself (which is to say, as past) or imagined (or rather, as future), but it is never lived in the present." Yes, it is possible to be consumed by nostalgia for a life one has never lived.

In Search of Lost Time

The past nurtures every form of nostalgia. There is no nostalgia except in the shadow of memory, in particular of the memory of things lived, and every recuperation of moods, situations, places that have given our lives meaning is nothing but an image of and metaphor for nostalgia. Those extraordinary pages that Marcel Proust devotes in the first chapter of his unforgettable book to Combray, where his childhood takes place—are they not, indeed, fed by nostalgia? I would like to quote certain passages that speak to us of childhood, of the early days of adolescence, and that submerge us in the depths of a generative nostalgia that reanimates the past and salvages a present consumed by restlessness and melancholy. But how do we revive the embers of the past? This great novel of time and memory, but also of nostalgia, offers us something of an answer. "It is the same with our past. It is a waste of effort for us to try to summon it, all the exertions of our intelligence are useless," and in Combray the past was reborn following unpredictable paths. "For many years, already, everything about Combray that was not the theater and drama of my bedtime had ceased to exist for me, when one day in winter, as I returned home, my mother, seeing that I was cold, suggested that, contrary to my habit, I have a little tea. I refused at first and then, I do not know why, changed my mind. She sent for one of those squat, plump cakes called petites madeleines that look as though they have been molded in the grooved valve of a scallop shell. And soon, mechanically, oppressed by the gloomy day and the prospect of another sad day to follow, I carried to my lips a spoonful of the tea in which I had let soften a bit of madeleine. But at the very instant when the mouthful of tea mixed with cake crumbs touched my palate, I quivered, attentive to the extraordinary thing that was happening inside me. A delicious pleasure had invaded me, isolated me, without my having any notion as to its cause. It had immediately rendered the vicissitudes of life unimportant to me, its disasters innocuous, its brevity illusory, acting in the same way that love acts, by filling me with a precious essence: or rather this essence was not merely inside me, it was me. I had ceased to feel mediocre, contingent, mortal."

If nostalgia is the evocation of a past full of light and hope, how can we not recognize it in this memory that is magical yet so quickly extinguished, and how do we make it rise back up again from the shadows? All at once, it reappears on its own. "That taste was the taste of the little piece of madeleine which on Sunday mornings at Combray (because that day I did not go out before it was time for Mass), when I went to say good morning to her in her bedroom, my aunt Léonie would give me after dipping it in her infusion of tea or lime blossom. The sight of the little madeleine had not reminded me of anything before I tasted it; perhaps because I had often seen them since, without eating them, on the shelves of the pastry shops, and their image had therefore left those days of Combray and attached itself to others more recent; perhaps because of these recollections abandoned so long outside my memory, nothing survived, everything had come apart; the forms and the form, too, of the little shell made of cake, so fatly sensual within its severe and pious pleating—had been destroyed, or, still half asleep, had lost the force of expansion that would have allowed them to rejoin my consciousness."

And having recognized the taste of this piece of madeleine soaked in tea, the long-lost landscape of childhood is reborn, as we see in this phantasmagoric image: "And as in that game enjoyed by the Japanese in which they fill a porcelain bowl with water and steep in it little pieces of paper until then indistinct which, the moment they are immersed, stretch and twist, assume colors and distinctive shapes, become flowers, houses, human figures, firm and recognizable, so now all the flowers in our garden and in M. Swann's park, and the water lilies of the Vivonne, and the good people of the village and their little dwellings and the church and all of Combray and its surroundings, all of this which is acquiring form and solidity, emerged, town and gardens alike, from my cup of tea."

These are delicate pages that have accompanied me throughout my life and that I continue to read along with countless others in Proust's grand novel of memory and nostalgia, especially when my days pass in the midst of tasks that dull them and empty them of meaning. They are pages that confront us with the endless horizons of a nostalgia that permits us to recover the past in its brilliance and its hope, its illusions and dreams, joining the past of experiences lived long ago with the present and above all with the future. There is no future, there is no horizon of hope, that does not derive from the past, from the hopes we've dreamed of that have left their trace on the present and future. Nostalgia is, in other words, the matrix of hope.

And Still, the Mystery of Childhood

Thus George Bernanos describes the passage from childhood to adolescence in his *The Carmelites*, in pages that glow with mysterious beauty. No writer has spoken of childhood with greater emotion or depth than Bernanos, as concludes Max Milner, who has devoted an entire book to him, one that remains relevant today, and its reflections are relevant here. Childhood, in

Bernanos, does not belong to the past, and when he looks back on childhood, it is not to revive a reality, which has the fascination of something annulled, but to turn his attention to that part of childhood that remains perpetually active. Childhood continues to be lived inside us, it is not expunged so long as we teach ourselves to listen to its secret voices, and Bernanos claimed he was always in dialogue with childhood, which was his eternal interlocutor, and to which he intended to remain faithful to the end. Not only that, but, in the moment of writing, Bernanos claimed, childhood was reborn within him, and the characters of his wonderful novels had already been prefigured in those early years. All that was good in his books came from long ago, from the magical wellspring of his youth and adolescence.

And I would be remiss not to mention the tenderness and grace, the gentleness and extreme sensitivity of two of the most fascinating and unforgettable Carmelite female figures who animate the dialogues, Blanche de la Force and Constance de Saint-Denis: both of them young, each different in their psychology, but so kindred in their nostalgia for childhood and their hope. The mortal anguish, the anguish of life and death, that characterized the life of Blanche de la Force, the kind and fragile protagonist of the dialogues, was overwhelmed by the hope that allowed her to accept death without fear. Hope never abandoned Constance de Saint-Denis in life or death: eternally suffused with the light of grace, never touched by the shadows of anguish, not even by the anguish of death. The two of them united in life and in death by a common fate, that of saving from the unceasing flow of time, of clock time and of lived time, the overlapping period of childhood and early adolescence. Bernanos's thinking about childhood, about its importance in his life and work, takes shape with arcane splendor, with shadow and light, in these two young Carmelite nuns. Their words, their indescribable compassion, are brightened by the glow of childhood, its lightness and airy luminosity, and it is hard to overlook their emotional resonances, which fill the soul of whoever reads these dialogues with an intelligence of the heart; and the heart's reason bring us far closer to the mystery of living and dying than the reasoning of the mind. What leads me to say all this, what leads me to speak of childhood as the matrix of the souls of Blanche de la Force and Constance de Saint-Denis? Of course, it is Bernanos's words, but above all, it is the ineffable lightness of his words that describe his subjects in a stage of life that is radically distant from all gravity (the gravity which Simone Weil opposes to grace in her marvelous texts) and from all personal prejudice, devoted simply to sympathetic listening and generosity, to simplicity, to self-sacrifice. These are the enigmatic connotations that Georges Bernanos assigned to childhood, dreamt and relived in its transparency and its splendors. Yes, I read and reread these dialogues, in which childhood, a silent and arcane subject, is renewed in its integral and mysterious charm.

The Fragility of Childhood

Fragility is the watchword of childhood. It embodies its various emotional manifestations, it seals its liquid boundaries with other life stages, with youth and every other age. There are words and modes that, perhaps in part due to their musicality, survive the passage of time intact, and are endowed with a high and even frenetic semantic density; fragility is one of these: lying at the root of an infinity of other emotional experiences. The fragility of childhood and adolescence possess modes of expression distinct from those present in other periods of life, even if they remain as an existential background. Nostalgia for childhood is not only nostalgia for a life open to infinite hopes; it is also a nostalgia for tenderness, for shelter, for compassion, for love, all of which were there alongside our fragility, only to run the risk of withering with the passage of years. We cannot forget these parts of childhood described by Dostoevsky, by Leopardi, by Proust, by Rilke, in stunning words and images, and they enable us to grasp it in its essential aspects.

The fragility of childhood, and in particular the fragility that comes with pain, is described in Andrea Bajani's beautiful novel, *One Good Thing in The World*, from which I would like to quote a few passages that speak of this delicacy and sensitivity. "There once was a boy who had a pain he never wanted to separate from. He took it with him everywhere, crossing town with it every morning on his way to school. When he got to class, the pain would curl up at his feet, and for five hours it didn't move an inch. At recess, the boy would carry it with him to the playground, and on his way home, he'd cross town the opposite way with the pain beside him." The striking clarity of this description plunges us directly into the burning fire of a fragility that runs throughout the book. Take the boy's walk and his pain on the roadside: "And every time they returned home, the boy would shut himself up in the only place he felt safe, but it wasn't a place, it was a feeling, and the feeling was called nostalgia," and further: "The boy had all the keys to that feeling. Its door was the only one his father and mother couldn't open. It was in there that the past, with all its amplified beauty, took the little boy in. The boy spent most of his time inside that feeling." And then: "In nostalgia, he was always happy, because everything had already happened and he didn't have anything to be afraid of. All it took to be happy, the boy thought, was never leaving that place he had unlocked. Happiness, he told himself, walking on the red rug and looking out the window, was locking away the good things that had happened. Growing up with what he had lived through, and then not living anymore. When he thought this, the boy would stroke his pain and finally feel happy. And of all things, that was the saddest of all."

What makes this novel a moving testimony to pain and fragility, to growth and the stirrings of love, the searing nostalgia for the hours that come and go unceasingly in a child's life? Of course, there is the delicacy of the description and the images, the poetic intensity that flows enchantingly across the pages, the intense and rarefied emotional resonance the narration sparks in us, the analogies gradually drawn between the fragility of childhood and the fragility of other periods of life; the metaphor of pain, represented as a gentle puppy the child converses with and which we are not easily in touch with once we are no longer children. But the book also invites us to walk down the mysterious path to interiority, which not seldom we lack the time or willingness to explore: distracted by a thousand mundane tasks that don't allow us the time to meditate on the values that come with childhood and that are forgotten or ignored in adulthood, at an ever-increasing pace and more radically, we are lost in a present that doesn't know how to look at the past or how to project itself into the future. A brief, elusive novel that leaves an indelible mark on our memory, and in a different way, to be sure, from those great writers I cited earlier, but that nonetheless compels us to reflect on the defenseless fragility and the secret pain of not a few children, who nowadays are not always kept close, nor listened to with the necessary compassion and patience that are so easily dissipated by haste and inattention, not unlike a love that is inadequate if not accompanied by that attention that Simone Weil calls tantamount to prayer. A novel that invites us, like all great works about childhood and youth, to think of the words and actions that open young hearts to hope.

In Dialogue With Childhood

How, then, can we not recognize the psychological and human importance of rethinking our own childhood, reliving it on the wings of nostalgia as we gradually become distant from it, without forgetting? This permits us not only to maintain a dialogue with our own childhood, with the emotional resonances that dialogue awakens in us, but also to enter into dialogue with the emotions, the expectations, and the hopes of children, in particular with their fragility and their pain. We should always be in dialogue with their pain in particular, the bitter pain of their bodies and their spirits, and we should be aware of the importance of our words and even our way of looking in the way their exhausted fragility is received and understood. How do we approach a child who is unwell, a sick child, a gravely ill child who requires an exemplary sensitivity to grasp the meaning of their tears and their desire for help? This is a question of our approach to understanding, or at least intuiting, what their visible and invisible wounds are, their anxieties, their sources of nostalgia. A child's illness, a child's suffering, confront us with a dual asymmetry, between the healer and the person who requires healing, and, more profoundly, between child and adult. It is never easy, and perhaps not always possible, to diminish or mend this asymmetry. But one thing is necessary: that we adults be capable of reviving the emotions, anxieties, sorrows, desires, hopes, fragility, and nostalgia that followed us through our youth. We will be able to do this so long as we do not eschew the habit of being aware, or trying to be aware, of what is hidden, of what is shifting, inside us, in our inner abysses, what lay there in our youth when we were unwell, when we were devoured by fragility, by loneliness, by pain, by nostalgia for bygone happiness, and the time of that affliction seemed to never pass.

The previous quotes from the texts of Dostoevsky, Leopardi, Rilke, Bernanos, and Andrea Bajani are meant to invite each of us to reflect on our past, on the experiences that we were able to have in our childhood, to fan the flame of their memory, to follow their mysterious trail. But when we are speaking with a child, especially with a sick child, our expression is of utmost importance: the measure of brightness and darkness, warmth and coolness, sparks and hollows, fears and anxieties, passion and indifference contained in our gaze. Speaking to or treating a child, we cannot but think of the importance of gentle and welcoming looks, accompanied by the hint of a smile (to add a thread, as Leopardi put it, to the short fabric of our life), that demonstrate listening, human closeness, emotional engagement, and care? There are times in our childhood when a person looks at us and it gives us joy and delight, serenity and hope, and that nostalgia draws forth from memory like kites flying up in the sky, as in Giovanni Pascoli's poetry, enigmatic and shot through with death; and there are other times when a look gives rise to sorrow and torment, to uncertainty and fear, to loneliness and pain in body and soul, thus subduing or extinguishing hope; and without hope, it is painful, exhausting, and sometimes impossible to live. Those are the looks we must remember, and we should select and summon those looks that have opened our hearts to hope.

A Nameless Nostalgia

A poignant image of nostalgia occurs in "A Vision," a poem by Hugo von Hofmannsthal, who in his adolescence composed poetry of unimaginable beauty, rekindled by the glow of childhood. Allow me to quote him here:

> The valley with a silver-grayish mist
> Of twilight was o 'e r brimmed, as when the moon
> Filters through clouds. And yet it was not night.
> In the silver-grayish mist of yon dark valley
> My twilight-shimmering thoughts were wholly
>   blended;
> Softly I sank into the shifting depths
> Of that transparent sea—and left this life.
> What wondrous flowers bloomed about me there
> With darkly glowing chalices!—dim thickets
> Transfused with streams of reddish-yellow light,
> Warm as a glowing topaz . And the vale
> Was filled with deep vibrating harmony
> Of melancholy music. Then I knew—
> Though how , I comprehend not—yet I knew
> That this was Death; Death was transformed to
>   music,
> Mightily yearning, sweet, and darkly glowing,
> Akin to deepest melancholy.
>   Yet—
> How strange! a sort of homesickness for life
> Wept silently within my soul, it wept

As one may weep when on a towering ship,
That drives toward evening with gigantic sails
Across the dark-blue waves, he passes by
A town, his native town. He sees before him
The streets, he hears the fountains gush, he breathes
The scent of lilac-bushes; on the bank
He sees himself a child with childish eyes
Anxious and almost weeping, sees a light
Through the wide window burning in his room.
But the huge vessel bears him ever on,
Silently speeding o'er the dark- blue waves
With giant sails of yellow, strangely shaped.

These images of nostalgia, a nostalgia that emerges from the boundless distances of childhood, shimmer in this poetry with esoteric allusivity, sparking ineffable responses in the soul. We cannot live without expectation or hope, yet we cannot live without nostalgia, either—without retracing the paths that take us back into the past, to the shadowy horizons of those memories that give life meaning. And what might this meaning be without nostalgia, without the memory that makes nostalgia possible, the memory which restores and reunites past, present, and future in their infinite circularity? Claudio Magris has spoken movingly about this poem and the impressions of childhood that radiate in it: "Modern poetry is often nostalgia for life: not for a specific and definable form of it whose absence is lamented, nor for some possession whose lack leaves us in pain and unhappy, but nostalgia for life itself, as though that itself were absent. 'There wept a mute and names / regret in me for life,' a line of Hofmannsthal says, and he compares this regret to the melancholy of one passing the city of his birth aboard a ship, seeing the familiar streets and gardens of his childhood and himself as a boy on the edge of town; he wants to respond to a light that greets him from a window, but the ship takes him further and further away." And finally: "In this image, life, which cannot be entered into, seems lost in the past rather than in the future, but it is always an absence, because regret is not directed at that boy's existence—that of the author himself as a boy—in those gardens, but at an existence that never was, a plenitude of meaning and happiness that a child can only expect and whose absence an adult can only regret."

The Fragile Beauty of Nature

Not only does the nostalgia for childhood exist, but also nostalgia for the beauty of nature that is so fragile as to be a source of pain. An evocative testimony thereto is the brief essay "Transience" by Sigmund Freud: "Not long ago I went on a summer walk through a smiling countryside in the company of a taciturn friend and of a young but already famous poet. The poet admired the beauty of the scene around us but felt no joy in it. He was disturbed by the thought that all this beauty was fated to extinction, that it would vanish with the winter, like all human beauty and all the beauty and splendor that men have created or may create. All that he would else have loved and admired seemed to him to be shorn of its worth by the transience which was its doom."

(In August of 1913, Freud spent his summer holiday in the Dolomites, but the identity of the person who accompanied him on his walk is unknown, though we cannot exclude the possibility that the young poet was Rainer Maria Rilke).

What does Freud tell us about the sorrow and the painful nostalgia of the young poet and the friend who was with them? "The proneness to decay of all that is beautiful and perfect can, as we know, give rise to two different impulses in the mind. The one leads to the aching despondency felt by the young poet, while the other leads to rebellion against the fact asserted. No! it is impossible that all this loveliness of Nature and Art, of the world of our sensations and of the world without, will really fade away into nothing. It would be too senseless and too presumptuous to believe it. Somehow or other this loveliness must be able to persist and to escape all the powers of destruction." Freud continues: "It was incomprehensible, I declared, that the thought of the transience of beauty should interfere with our joy in it. As regards the beauty of Nature, each time it is destroyed by winter it comes again next year, so that in relation to the length of our lives it can in fact be regarded as eternal. The beauty of the human form and face vanish for ever in the course of our own lives, but their evanescence only lends them a fresh charm. A flower that blossoms only for a single night does not seem to us on that account less lovely." Freud's considerations were not shared by the young poet, nor by the friend who was with them; and for this reason, he writes: "My failure led me to infer that some powerful emotional factor was at work which was disturbing their judgement, and I believed later that I had discovered what it was. What spoilt their enjoyment of beauty must have been a revolt in their minds against mourning. The idea that all this beauty was transient was giving these two sensitive minds a foretaste of mourning over its decease; and, since the mind instinctively recoils from anything that is painful, they felt their enjoyment of beauty interfered with by thoughts of its transience."

These are his conclusions, but regardless, Freud knew how splendidly to describe the moods, the emotions, the vicissitudes of the spirit, the painful nostalgia (how can we not hear its faint echo in ourselves as well?) of the young poet and their common friend at the thought of the fragility and precarity of life, its transience and its rapid withering, its grace and its gravity. Yes, *sunt lacrimae rerum*, and how shall we ever wipe them away?

We Cannot Live Without Nostalgia

We cannot live without nostalgia: this is the intense, affecting testimony contained in the words of Etty Hillesum's diary, a book one never stops reading. She wrote these words on September 17, 1942 in Amsterdam, the city of her birth, where she managed to return briefly from Westerbork concentration camp, and from where, a year later, she was sent to die in Auschwitz with her parents and one of her brothers, Mischa, a talented young pianist. "I so wish I could put it all into words. Those two months behind barbed wire have been the two richest and most intense months of my life, in which my highest values were so deeply confirmed. I have learned to love Westerbork. Yet when I fell asleep on my narrow plank bed there, what I dreamed of was the desk behind which I now sit and write. 'I am so grateful to You, God, for having made my life so rich, but no matter where You place me, I always long for that desk of mine.' But it does make life rather difficult and hard at times. It's now past 10:30, the time when they turn out the lights in the barracks, and when I myself must turn in." Life's nostalgias are uncountable: they emerge, they fade and disappear, and precipitously reappear in the most diverse settings. A few days later, on September 22, Etty Hillesium feels nostalgia for Westerbork, and wonders: "How is it that this stretch of heathland surrounded by barbed wire, through which so much human misery has flooded, nevertheless remains inscribed in my memory as something almost lovely? How is it that my spirit, far from being oppressed, seemed to grow lighter and brighter there? It is because I read the signs of the times and they did not seem meaningless to me. Surrounded by my writers and poets and the flowers on my desk, I loved life. And there among the barracks, full of hunted and persecuted people, I found confirmation of my love of life. Life in those drafty barracks was no other than life in this protected, peaceful room." And her nostalgia for the concentration camp reemerges in these words: "How can I draw this small village of barracks between heath and sky with a few rapid, delicate, and yet powerful, strokes of the pen? And how can I let others see the many inmates, who have to be deciphered like hieroglyphs, stroke by stroke, until they finally form one great readable and comprehensible whole?"

In the tumultuous passing of years, we are devoured not only by nostalgia for childhood and adolescence, for youth and adulthood, but also by the nostalgias that descend upon us, within each season of our lives, in different places, just as with Etty Hillesium, who felt nostalgia for her own home *and* at the same time for the barracks of Westerbork concentration camp. This, again, occurs only if we never tire of figuring out and analyzing our thoughts and our emotions, our expectations and our hopes, because it is on these, endlessly, that nostalgia feeds, helping us to once again set down those paths that lead inside ourselves. Nostalgia leads us to a knowledge of the hidden and secret regions of our past, and in revealing our past errors and faults, enables us to avoid them in the future, which broadens nostalgia's ethical boundaries. Yes, everything is connected, as Friedrich Hölderlin wrote in deep and stirring words, and in nostalgia, the past, present, and future are interwoven in Augustinian circularity. Nostalgia is truly inside us, however difficult it is to recognize in its subtle psychological and interpersonal manifestations.

Without a Homeland

To flee one's native land, Africa in particular, as so many people have done to escape abominable living conditions not so far from those experienced by Etty Hillesium, brings with it an infinite pain that is attested to by the faces shown on television, whose despair is impossible not to recognize. If in exile—the choice, more or less voluntary, to live in another country—nostalgia is a constant and friendly travel companion, as María Zambrano describes in her wonderful essays, it is less so in the desperate flight from one's homeland. There is no assurance of a humane welcome when one reaches one's destination; and then, is it possible to feel nostalgia from the places one has run away from in the hope of a tranquil life? These people we see on our television screens and come across in our cities, united by unspeakable, inseparable sufferings of body and soul—how can we not feel compelled to shelter them in their wounded humanity, which may be, though we cannot say whether or how much, wracked with nostalgia and regrets that horribly intensify their pain and despair?

The causes of these painful migrations today are poverty, violence, and encroaching death. People leave on boats or ships, the threat of shipwreck ever-present, the numerous heartrending cases at times leaving us in the rut of arid indifference. But for those who manage to reach Europe safely, how can we ignore the wounds in their souls, from the painful the loss of their homeland and yearning for their families who have not always followed in their migration? We should be capable of receiving and sharing in their anguish and sorrow, their suffering and despair, and of understanding the loneliness and the bite of nostalgia in such fragile existences, existences exposed to humiliations of all sort, like those coming from Africa and trying to reach our shores in search of lost peace. These are wounded existences that call for concrete actions, but also silent words that will attest that we are listening, that will attest to our solidarity, and fundamentally, to our hopes: something quite difficult, but necessary nonetheless. Hope is only granted to the hopeless: these arcane, unforgettable words of Walter Benjamin are ones we should never forget.

Nostalgia for Africa

I don't know how, or whether, no matter what they go through, people who immigrate to Europe still long for their homeland or hope for its conflicts and violence to come to an end. A nostalgia for Africa, for African peoples, is certainly felt by the missionaries and volunteers who wish to return there after coming back to Italy, fascinated by the kindness of the African people who retain their dignity even in the most devastating and tragic conditions. Is there an unbreachable contradiction between the flight from Africa and the nostalgia for it? These thoughts inevitably resurface every time we read Karen Blixen's extraordinary pages about an Africa that no longer exists but lives on in her unforgettable landscapes, especially in the immense humanity and enduring tenderness of the men and women in her books. Nostalgia for Africa consumed the great Danish author's life and filled it with generosity and solidarity, passion and creativity, love and with death. Her book *Out of Africa* possesses a strange beauty that persists in our memory, recalling an Africa still tranquil and kind. A book which, at least in a certain stage of our lives, fills us with an impossible nostalgia, a longing to know Karen Blixen's Africa in its human and psychological aspects which have essentially remained alive, as we know from those missionaries and volunteers, in the hearts of those Africans *not* oppressed by unspeakable violence. It is a book that loses nothing of its emotional resonance and beauty in Sydney Pollack's cinematic adaptation, which features the splendid acting of Robert Redford and particularly Meryl Streep, who embodies Karen Blixen's fervor and passion, her dedication and her boundless nostalgia for an Africa that had taken root in her soul. The film introduces us to the weary beauty of its countryside, its colors, its music, and fosters our nostalgia for a time that will never again be what it once was. A film I felt it proper to mention here, because even now, it tells us something about Africa, that land today torn apart by conflict and war, its nature and its lifeways turned upside down, a land that fills us with nostalgia for the Africa of yore, albeit without forgetting the cruel colonialism of the past.

Nostalgia as a Metaphor for Life

Nostalgia is a part of life, as is memory, which feeds into nostalgia with recollections that we should never forget, recollections that help us to live. There is no life immune to the now bright, now shaded paths of nostalgia and its sister emotions of melancholy, sorrow, regret, spiritual pain, wounded joy and delight—and many are the forms nostalgia assumes in the different stages of our lives. To seek emotions, lost emotions—and nostalgia is the emblematic testament to this—is the task of all who would know the boundless regions of interiority and the emotions that form part of it. We ought not live without constantly reflecting on the story of our life, the past that constitutes it that nostalgia allows us to revive, things we could have done and did not, missed opportunities, all the possibilities still ahead of us, and finally, the reasons for our nostalgia and our regrets. Not only is it possible, it is common to want to flee from experience and awareness of what we once were and are now.

Nostalgia is founded on memory, which is its source. If that memory is flawed or damaged by the wounds that illness or misfortune bring, then how will we recognize the traces of nostalgia in ourselves? Naturally, it is from emotional memory, from experiential memory, that nostalgia springs, not from rational memory, the memory of names and numbers, which has nothing to do with the emotional sort; and any reflection on the endless theme of memory, admirably explored by Saint Augustine in his *Confessions*, must keep its complex and problematic nature constantly in mind.

Nostalgia as a Cause of Illness

Nostalgia has unfolded in the course of these pages of mine as mood, as *Stimmung*, as an emotional experience, as a sentiment, as a form of life, as desire, as *le douceur du foyer* (as Jean Starobinski tells us Baudelaire called it), as a shade of memory, and deep down, as the recovery of events from the past, a past at once far away and close, misplaced, as it were, but not lost forever. This is the spontaneous and immediate image that is born in us, in each of us, when we think of nostalgia, and when we relive it in our emotional and relational life. But now, I would like to examine a different image of nostalgia, one painful and searing in its effects, one that accompanies depression and anguish, melancholy, and illness of the spirit and perhaps of the body, too. Naturally, in this altered phenomenology of nostalgia, the way we experience time doesn't change, but its emotional context does: no longer sweet and bright, it is now bitter and dark. And this has been the original image of nostalgia.

The history of medicine tells us how nostalgia, the nostalgia for a lost homeland, was constituted as a morbid condition that appeared in young Swiss soldiers sent off to places far from home. This was described by Johannes Hofer in his doctoral dissertation, which brought nostalgia back into the medical arena, and secondarily into the psychiatric one. At this point, I would like to turn briefly to this subject, which even now retains a certain level of clinical interest. Nostalgia, which throughout the history of medicine was defined a malady, was eventually withdrawn from clinical medical texts, but endured in psychiatric literature up through the early twentieth century. Jean Starobinski considers this subject: "Why, Johannes Hofer asked himself, are young Swiss people so frequently inclined to nostalgia when they find themselves in another country? Undoubtedly, because many of them have never left their family home, because they have never been to a foreign land. And so they struggle to forget the care their mother lavished on them. They miss the soup they customarily had for breakfast, the fine milk of their valleys, and perhaps even the freedom they enjoyed in their homeland... The contemporary psychologist must be grateful to Johannes Hofer for having emphasized so early the role of 'affective deficiency'; the regretful yearning for childhood, for 'oral satisfactions,' and for maternal care."

As Starobinski tells us, Johannes Hofer rightly traces nostalgia back to its emotional roots, but also to its connections to solitude, affective deficiencies, the loss of familial relations, and the duties of work, grasping, at least in part, its complex psychological and social resonances. Today, the word *nostalgia* has disappeared from medical and psychiatric writings, even if it may be the cause of a particular form of depression, as I will discuss next, but its indelible semantic arc as a form of emotional life has not been, in all cases, suppressed, but has emerged as the search for the meaning of things that occurred in the past, and that live on, subdued and sometimes hidden within us, in the abysses of our memory and our inner life. I would like now to offer an emblematic psychopathological and clinical testimony of this depression that will also highlight its human dimension.

Nostalgia for Home

The thematic traces of nostalgia as an illness, above all as depression, can be glimpsed even today if one does not weary of listening to patients with one eye on the clock, setting aside the impulse to catalogue their psychological disturbances and classify them according to the cold definitions of symptomatology. If we do this, we may encounter a psychiatric patient like Costanza, for whom moving house brought on a depression. What has occurred in a case such as this? Leaving our "old house" to go live in another bigger and nicer one gradually brings on the burning desire to go back to the one before, a place filled with memories and silences, stories, inner life. It is not the distance between one house and another that causes this nostalgia and disquiet: we can move without leaving the city where we live and nonetheless be afflicted with crippling nostalgia. Just the loss of one's roots and native land can cause depression, a change of dwelling can bring about the same: both are marked by sadness, desolation, yearning, and a sense of loss. A change of home triggered in Costanza a dark affliction, a distaste for life, utter sorrow, which developed into a pathological depression that was stemmed and finally resolved with antidepressants. The home she lived in for many years contained the story of Costanza's life, all its joys and sufferings, expectations and hopes, pains and nostalgia, and this place was truly part of her life. Not only its interiors, the language of familiar objects, books, but also the exterior spaces, the landscape that the windows looked out upon—all this articulated the rhythms and significance of her days. Be it beautiful or ugly, a dwelling—when it is *lived*—creates an entire ecosystem of security, a tacit dialogue between people and things. And such must have been Costanza's house, if I think back on what she told me about her house, the feeling and nostalgic tenderness of her words; at any rate, she felt and experienced the spaces of her *new* house as uncomfortably quiet and still, whereas her spatial concept of the *old* house was free-flowing, moving from interior to exterior, from outside back in. Yet other sensations, too, animated the patient's wounded soul.

In the new house, it was impossible to plant flowers and keep them alive, those fragile and ethereal presences that warmed her former home and were a touchstone of Costanza's expressions of nostalgia. "The flowers gave our house a touch of grace, even though it wasn't very nice." (Trakl's blue flowers that echo in the yellowed stone, but also the flowers that the desolate heart of Gérard de Nerval loved so: how much luminosity, how much lightness, how much graceful phosphorescence there is in flowers). These are fragile and volatile subjects, ungraspable like sand between one's fingers, crepuscular and nostalgic, but there is another possible nostalgia in looks and gestures, in smiles and tears, in landscapes, that gradually withdraws in space but remains present in memory. These are motifs nurtured by a mysterious, luminous life and feed the soul with expectations and hopes; and on these motifs it is possible to live and die, and the wounds of the soul can cut far deeper than the wounds of the body. These motifs resurface in all their human and clinical manifestations when psychiatry encounters depressive episodes like Costanza's, which slowly self-perpetuate in the wake of an impalpable but nonetheless rending nostalgia, accompanied by worsening sorrow and anguish.

Time

There is no psychological or human experience unrelated to the presence of time: not only clock time, hourglass time, world time, which measures that which comes into the present and marks the hours equally within us, but also inner time, subjective time, lived time, the time that extends from the present into the past and projects itself into the future, the time that allows us to live in a way distinct from the simple passing of hours. An hour of time, when we are tired or sad, can be long, even interminable, but it may be fluid and fast when we are content or excited. Our moods and emotions influence our perceptions of time, and this in turn is mirrored in the way we relate to others. When we are waiting for something or someone, when pain falls upon us, when we are bored and life seems to be without meaning, time—inner time—refuses to pass, and we keep looking at the clock, which seems to move with extraordinary slowness. But when we are pleased, or for example, reading a book that interests us, time flows so quickly that we don't notice. As for inner time, lived time, we manage to be aware of it, I must stress, only when following the path that leads into the unfathomable abysses of our inner selves. To quote Saint Augustine's *Confessions*, which contains marvelous reflections on time that we all know yet may have forgotten: "For what is time? Who can easily and briefly explain it? Who can even comprehend it in thought or put the answer into words? Yet is it not true that in conversation we refer to nothing more familiarly or knowingly than time? And surely we understand it when we speak of it; we understand it also when we hear another speak of it. What, then, is time? If no one asks me, I know what it is. If I wish to explain it to him who asks me, I do not know. Yet I say with confidence that I know that if nothing passed away, there would be no past time; and if nothing were still coming, there would be no future time; and if there were nothing at all, there would be no present time. But, then, how is it that there are the two times, past and future, when even the past is now no longer and the future is now not yet? But if the present were always present, and did not pass into past time, it obviously would not be time but eternity. If, then, time present—if it be time—comes into existence only because it passes into time past, how can we say that even this is, since the cause of its being is that it will cease to be?"

Saint Augustine responds to these questions saying that the present, past, and future are dimensions of the soul, which continually encroach upon one other: "But even now it is manifest and clear that there are neither times future nor times past. Thus it is not properly said that there are three times, past, present, and future. Perhaps it might be said rightly that there are three times: a time present of things past; a time present of things present; and a time present of things future. For these three do coexist somehow in the soul, for otherwise I could not see them. The time present of things past is memory; the time present of things present is direct experience; the time present of things future is expectation. If we are allowed to speak of these things so, I see three times, and I grant that there are three. Let it still be said, then, as our misapplied custom has it: 'There are three times, past, present, and future.' I shall not be troubled by it, nor argue, nor object—always provided that what is said is understood, so that neither the future nor the past is said to exist now."

Augustine's reflections on time, on the subjective experience of time, marked a radical and revolutionary turn in the history of philosophical and psychopathological thinking about time, tracing it back to its ineluctable inner dimension.

The Time of Nostalgia

The time of nostalgia is the past, the uninterrupted passage from the present to the past, and so, does the future have nothing to do with nostalgia? At the beginning of a remarkable article on nostalgia, Chiara Mirabelli writes that the time of nostalgia implicates not only the past, but also the future: "It includes that which no longer is and that which could be in the tension of time that opens toward the present." And then: "Every origin contains its goal: and to imagine our future differently, to open what was in our past, even our remote past, to new directions, redefines our very origins. It changes the shape of those "life writings" found in the etymological roots of the word 'autobiography.' 'Aching to return' is something we can interpret not only as the pain we feel because we are unable to return, but also as the necessary reworking of what was painful in our past, restoring dynamism to both past and present." These are innovative concepts: nostalgia is not only the spark of a feeling that conjures up both remote and recent experiences from the past, missing or lost, obscure or luminous, and that helps us to reconsider them within their horizons of meaning, perhaps to allow them to be reconstituted and revived, giving them a future. This broadens the human and psychological significance of nostalgia, nostalgia in the many forms it takes in our lives, in particular the value of the experiences of youth, those embers that have not burned out entirely and may reignite and immerse themselves creatively once more, in the story of each of our lives. And so nostalgia is the rediscovery of a past that is reborn as open possibility, neither lost definitively nor erased from our personal history.

In this way, in nostalgia, in the time of nostalgia, past, present, and future weave together: whether moving from an originary experience of desire, the desire for a return from the present, a present of pain, to a past that gradually grows clearer in its outlines, its lights and shadows, its illusions and disillusions, its emotional distances and proximities, but also in its expectations and its hopes of recovery, rebirth, transcendence, futurity. The spur that sets in motion to the infinite movement of nostalgia, of the memories it is nourished on, is discontent with that which appears in the present, in the ephemeral hours of the present, and the desire to get away from it, to put it between brackets, while searching for a lifeboat, a subconscious longing for a cure. Yes, nostalgia is healing: it is the coalescing of desires that have lost every horizon of meaning in the present and look to the past as a possible source of salvation.

What do these considerations tell us? One thing, above all: not experiencing nostalgia, not harboring the desires that give meaning to the vertiginous fleeing of time and the recovery of those values that were part of our youth, is not living, or at least not as it is recognizable in its horizons of meaning. True, the places and phases of life, the time to which the paths of nostalgia lead us, are, or at least can be, pleasant or painful, dark or bright, and either way, compel us to think back on mistakes made and good not done; and so nostalgia permits us to retrace the path, however long, of our lives, helping us recognize the things we should have done and the ones that we can still do, to rethink them and modify our actions as we realize them.

An Aside

Giorgio Agamben has recently written very interestingly on the subject of time, some of which I will quote here. "'I have such trust in the future that I only make plans in the past.' This phrase of by Ennio Flaiano—a writer whose jokes must be taken extremely seriously—contain a truth it is worth-while to reflect on. The future, like the crisis, is today one of the principal and most effective instruments of power. Whether this is waved before us like a menacing bogeyman (impoverishment and ecological disasters) or as a radiant future (in cloying progressivism), it is, in either case, a way of perpetuating the notion that we must exclusively orient our thoughts and our actions to it. In other words, we should put aside the past, which can't be changed and is anyway useless—or at most put away in a museum—and as for the present, we should only take an interest in it to the extent that it serves to prepare for the future."

But that isn't so: "Nothing could be more false: the only thing we possess and can know with any certainty is the past, while the present is, by defini-tion, difficult to grasp, and the future, which doesn't exist, can be made up out of whole cloth by any charlatan. In private life and in the public sphere, distrust those who offer you a future: such people almost always trying to entrap you or trick you. 'I shall not allow the shadow of the future,' writes Ivan Illich, 'to fall on the concepts with which I try to grasp what is and what has been.' And Benjamin has observed that in memories (which are different from the immobile archive of memory) we are actually acting on the past, in a certain way we make it possible again. Flaiano was right to suggest to us that we make plans for the past. Only an archeological investigation into the past can allow us to access the present, while one turned solely to the future dispossess us, as well as our past, of the present."

And finally: "You know that in both individual and collective life, the great mass of things lost, the wastage of the tiny, imperceptible events that we forget every day, is almost exterminated, and there is no archive and no memory that might safeguard them. What is left, that part of language and life that we salvage from ruin, has meaning only if it is intimately related to what is lost, if it stands somehow with what is lost, if it calls it by its name and responds in its name."

These reflections permit me to say, or at least to repeat, that in its way of looking, in its evocation of the past, that which happened in the past, the past of life, of our lives and in history, as an epiphany of the past, nostalgia leads us to fulfill the horizons of meaning, the ideals, that Agamben has illustrated. Yes, nostalgia, even when oriented toward drawing forth experiences we miss from our past, helps us not to be prisoners to a present and a past that instead ought always to be correlated with the past, with experiences from our past, with that inner history without which we are simply closed and isolated monads, incapable of meditation and reflection and lost in the contemplation of a rootless future. Without universalizing cognitive and ethical perspectives, nostalgia, the memories that it awakens from their stillness and their silence, revives the past still throbbing with life, as Walter Benjamin says in his unforgettable texts on memory and the fruitfulness of the past.

Nostalgia is Reborn from Memory

How is it even possible to talk about nostalgia, about an emotion so fragile and stubborn, so chameleonic and ungraspable, without anchoring it to the discourse concerning the boundless and problematic areas of memory as a premise for the birth and death of nostalgia? The path of awareness leads inward, toward the abysses of interiority, and from this splendid metaphor I would like to move again to grasp the meaning of the possible alliance between memory and interiority, memory and nostalgia, memory and lived time.

Memory is immersed in time, is born of the past and lives on the past, and from lived memory emerge continually the memories that feed nostalgia and are modified with changes in mood, changes in emotion, changes in situation, weaving together endlessly with the ways in which the future, life to come, is lived. Indeed, past is converted into future, and the content of nostalgia may be mirrored in the content of hope. Lived memory is emotional memory, memory as a site of inner experience, of emotions experienced in the past that still linger, and these have *absolutely nothing* to do with rational memory, the memory of names, numbers, objective events that unfold in mathematic and geometric memory along the course of time. From the vast quarters of lived memory emerge swarms of images and memories that are feverishly relived in the present, and that take on emotional and existential significance only if the intentional continuity of time is undisturbed, only if and when past, present, and future are woven together into a single unit.

And so, there is no lived memory except insofar as the past flows into the future: into hope. Memory, which lives on the past and in the past, and the expectation and hope that live on the future and in the future, are mysteriously anchored in each other; and from memory, from lived memory, recollections reemerge every time like herons drunk and sated on our nostalgia, which animates them and allows them to persist through time, radiating their influence toward the future, and more generally toward life. It is impossible to reflect on the vast confines of nostalgia, which is like a raft setting forth into the dark nights of the soul, if one ignores its uninterrupted interactions with memory.

In concerning itself with an emotional form of life such as nostalgia, psychiatry cannot but relate it to other forms of life, other psychic functions, and in particular to memory, if psychiatry is to be understood as a human and not only a natural science. And so, I find myself compelled to turn once again to Saint Augustine's immortal *Confessions*, to certain considerations of memory that remain startlingly modern. Only in the thematic context of time and memory is it possible to approach an understanding of nostalgia, of the emotional and existential incandescence that marks it, of the complex and problematic horizons that delimit it. It is so easy to trivialize the ethical and semantic foundations of nostalgia, treating it as a waste of time, a pointless and idle reverie, an obsessive rumination on things that happened in the past and that are pointless to linger on even for a second, as they are an obstacle to living a life freely open to the future, to all that is to come. The rejection of nostalgia mirrors the exaltation of a time that has only a present and future, but no past.

From the chapter of the *Confessions* devoted to memory, I would like to extract a few fragments that attest to its obscure foundations: "And I enter the fields and spacious halls of memory, where are stored as treasures the countless images that have been brought into them from all manner of things by the senses. There, in the memory, is likewise stored what we cogitate, either by enlarging or reducing our perceptions, or by altering one way or another those things which the senses have made contact with; and everything else that has been entrusted to it and stored up in it, which oblivion has not yet swallowed up and buried. When I go into this storehouse, I ask that what I want should be brought forth. Some things appear immediately, but others require to be searched for longer, and then dragged out, as it were, from some hidden recess." The nostalgia of his mysterious path brings forth images possessed with emotional tension and arcane fascination, and have resisted the oblivion of forgetting, which often devours even the most meaningful experiences of our lives if our inner fabric is fragile and frayed. Nostalgia, neglected and easily repressed, is like a light that illuminates the darkness and the gaps in the memory of what has been, what will not be again, and feeds on the passion of interiority.

Saint Augustine's words immerse us in the vortex of forgetting, the amnesia that strikes names and places, with almost unimaginable insights—but what does all this have to do with the pressing theme of nostalgia? I don't know, and yet it is possible to feel nostalgia for something that one knows how to define only in vague contours that become clearer in time. These are words that help psychiatry to face with the problem of amnesia.

"But what happens when the memory itself loses something, as when we forget anything and try to recall it? Where, finally, do we search, but in the memory itself? And there, if by chance one thing is offered for another, we refuse it until we meet with what we are looking for; and when we do, we recognize that this is it. But we could not do this unless we recognized it, nor could we have recognized it unless we remembered it. Yet we had indeed forgotten it. Perhaps the whole of it had not slipped out of our memory; but a part was retained by which the other lost part was sought for, because the memory realized that it was not operating as smoothly as usual and was being held up by the crippling of its habitual working; hence, it demanded the restoration of what was lacking."

On the Path

This book attempts to reassess the horizons of meaning of nostalgia, this mood, this form of life, this silent search for a future and for hope, along the mysterious path that leads to the boundless region of interiority. Nostalgia permits us to recover lost time and lost places, submerged memories, elusive hopes. We are a thousand miles away here from the notion of nostalgia as illness, a pointless waste of time, a distance from life and from social relations, a symptom of depression, of the loss of vital contact with life, as the arena of futile semantic conflict or of linguistic quarrels. Nostalgia has multiple forms of expression, but its thematic core persists despite the ravages of time, time that separates us from Johannes Hofer's groundbreaking thesis, because, in the semantic arc of nostalgia, there is something hidden that corresponds to an essential aspect of life.

I can do no better, in describing the emotional heights of nostalgia and its arcane semantics, that to turn again to poetry: to Emily Dickinson, to Giovanni Pascoli, to Paul Celan, each different from the other, each with a distinct mode of expression, but all of them witnesses to the chameleonic modes of being of nostalgia, not only nostalgia for youth but also for intense experiences lest they be lost forever. Not only this, but every book of my own that I have published has been in dialogue with madness (madness being the ill-starred sister of poetry, in the striking definition of the great German Romantic poet Clemens Brentano), and following the hermeneutic path of German- and Dutch-language psychiatry, has always been accompanied by literary quotations that offer a window, another point of view, onto the enigmas of wounded interiority and the emotions derive from it, which are the object, or rather, the subject, of psychiatry. It is a science that becomes inescapably human whenever it seeks—and how can it not?—to create interpersonal relations and institute communities of care which are, whenever possible, also communes of fate.

When Friends Die

The poetry of Emily Dickinson, so different from that of Leopardi, draws on a nostalgia born not only of lost adolescence, but of the diminishment, the death, of loved ones, and the fragile, ineffable grace of her imagination echoes even in this brief letter: "Dear friend. I send you a flower from my garden — Though it dies in reaching you, you will know it lived, when it left my hand — Hamlet wavered for all of us."

Her poetry is marked by the shadows of the burning bushes of memory that filled the silence of the solitude she lived in. Painful memories, rending memories, are reborn in the poem, "If Anybody's Friend Be Dead," which addresses the death of people close to the author; and the poem reevokes their fragile and heartwrenching gestures, their smiles, their ways of being. These are nuances of life that the subtlety and attention, the immediacy and the intuition of the inexpressible that Emily Dickinson captures in all their emblematic human significance. Of a beloved person who is no longer with us, we remember so many things with painful nostalgia, but especially their little gestures, their ways of moving, their ways of listening and smiling, and all these persist in our memory, which is racked with pain.

I would cite, however, another diaphanous Emily Dickinson poem here, on the nostalgia for death and dying: a poem brief as a breath and ungraspable as a dragonfly:

> The World – feels Dusty
> When We stop to Die –
> We want the Dew – then –
> Honors – taste dry –
>
> Flags – vex a Dying face –
> But the least Fan
> Stirred by a friend's Hand –
> Cools – like the Rain –
>
> Mine be the Ministry
> When thy Thirst comes –
> And Hybla Balms –
> Dews of Thessaly, to fetch –

These are brittle, painful words, immersed as always in an airy and subdued emotional atmosphere, that move us to rethink the most afflicting and untamed form of nostalgia, which is the nostalgia for death and dying, for ourselves as well as the loved ones who have left us behind.

The Kite

The poetry of Giovanni Pascoli is immersed in the calm and burning, silent and turbulent waters of a nostalgia infused with melancholy, which intertwine to form the basis of his lyrical imagination.

Among Pascoli's most intense and stirring poems is "The Kite," a painful and nostalgic journey back to the feverish age of adolescence.

> There's something new in the sun to-day – but no,
> More like something old: at this distance even
> I sense the violets starting to peep through
>
> Beside the Convent of the Capuchins,
> On the wood floor, between the stumps of oak
> Where dead leaves shilly-shally in the wind.
>
> A breath of mild air breathes, its little frolic
> Cajoles hard clods, combs the yielding grass
> Round country churches green up to the doorstep -

Air from another life and time and place,
Pale blue heavenly air that is holding up
A flotilla of white wings on the breeze –

The kites! Yes, it is! The kites! It's that morning
And there's no school and we've come trooping out
Among the briar hedges and the hawthorn.

The hedges bristled, shivered, spiky, stripped,
But autumn lingered in red clumps of berries
And spring in a few flowers, blooming white.

A robin hopped around the leafless branches.
In the ditch a lizard showed its darting head
Above dead leaves and vanished: a few scurries.

So now we take our stand, halt opposite
Urbino's windy hill: each scans the blue
And picks his spot to launch his long-tailed comet.

And there it hovers, flips, veers, dives askew,
Lifts again, goes with the wind until
It rises to loud cheers from us kids below.

It rises, and the hand is like a spool
Unspooling thread, the kite a thin-stemmed flower
Borne far away to flower again as windfall.

It rises and it carries ever higher
The longing in the breast and anxious feet
And gazing face and heart of the kite-flier.

Higher and higher until it's just a dot
Of brightness far, far up…But now a sudden
Crosswind and a scream…Whose scream was that?

Companions' voices rise to me unbidden
And familiar, still the same old chorus
Of sweet and high and hoarse. And there isn't,

My friends, one I don't recognize, and yes,
Of us all, you in particular, who droop your head
On your shoulder and avert your quiet face,

You, over whom I shed my tears and prayed,
You who were lucky to have seen the fallen
Only in the windfall of a kite.

You were very pale, I remember, but had grown
Red at the knees from kneeling on the floor -
Raw from all that praying night and morning.

And ah, were you not lucky to cross over
With confidence in your eyes, and in your arms
The plaything that of all things was most dear.

Gently, I well know, when the time comes
We die with our childhood clasped close to our breast
Like a flower in bloom that closes and reforms

Its petals into itself. O you, so young, the youngest
Of my dead, I too will soon go down into the clay
Where you sleep calmly, on your own, at rest.

Better to arrive there breathless, like a boy
Who has been racing up a hill,
Flushed and hot and soft, a boy at play,

Better to arrive there with a full
Head of blond hair, which spread cold on the pillow
As you mother combed it, wavy and beautiful,

Combed it slowly so as not to hurt you.

In the poem, Pascoli imagines himself as a boy, on a carefree day when he and his friends flew kites in the windy Urbino sky. The kites, ebullient with airy lightness, rise in the sky, only to fall back down to the earth and die. The happy memory of adolescence is entwined with bitter pain at a schoolmate's death , and in the flashback, nostalgia and sorrow, joy and unhealed wounds alternate in a dizzying lyrical dance. The poem tells us that to die young is sweeter than to live long, and this was the fate of his young companion. And it is impossible not to dwell on the weary tenderness (the fragility of words when they try to say the unsayable) of the last verse: where the mother combs the boy's hair gently so as not to hurt him, her now lifeless son. A mother's pain knows no limits.

The thematic sequences, light and digressive, fluid and colorful, unfold at the brink of a boundless nostalgia, and every time we read this poem, we are called to think again of our own adolescence: the joy and heartache, the expectations and hopes, some of them wounded forever. The phosphorescent, unforgettable image of nostalgia, its mystery, is mirrored in this poem, one of Pascoli's most excruciating, and one that it is hard to read and reread unmoved. The doubled image of nostalgia, as a source of levity and pain, reappears in luminous poignancy, and accompanied by bitter reflections on life, the meaning of life, which already in adolescence is filled lights and shadows that are impossible to escape.

This splendid poem permits us to grasp what nostalgia is in its most arcane and secret dimensions, dark and bright, painful and bittersweet.

Les adieux

To the poems of Emily Dickinson and Giovanni Pascoli, I would like to add one by the great, perhaps the greatest, German-language poet from the last century, Paul Celan, who knew in life the shadows of madness and who chose a death by drowning himself in the waters of the Seine.

Here is his poem, "Les adieux":

Silken moth of nostalgia:
Night drums in the calyx of the tulips…
And dying clouds are wine!

What will become of my blood now?

Dove and dew were life…

Dove and dew are death, too.

Ay, grasses, your stem of stars:
What is the wind that uproots you?

These silken moths of nostalgia are the incandescent, liquid metaphor in which floats this hermetic poem by Celan, who knows better than anyone how to painfully evidence lightness and phosphorescence, unpredictability and enigmaticness. As in all his poems, this contains chasms of obscurity that cannot be deciphered other than by following one's intuition, far from the glaring light of calculating reason, anchored rather in the rationale of the heart.

Nostalgia Rediscovered

Nostalgia, immersion in the unstill waters of our emotional life, is an experience that at times we seek, in defiance of habit and the distractions of our day-to-day life, and at times it resurfaces in an image, a letter, a book, a photo, a song, a landscape, a meeting, even a simple word. Nostalgia speaks to us of the tendency that arises in us all to imbue the past, our past experiences, with meaning, and not let it die. In particular, we see reborn the variously distant values of childhood and adolescence, which help free us, or try to, at least in part, from the traces left behind by the advancing years.

My wish for the present work on nostalgia is that it bear witness to the vast thematic horizons and the deep emotional and existential resonances that this phenomenon awakens within us, in the abysses of our interiority. Occasionally forgotten and trivialized, nostalgia helps us to live, to reconstruct lived time in its unitary circularity of past, present, and future, and to draw forth recollections of childhood, adolescence, youth, and other stages of life from our memory that strip off the rust of the feverish and fatal passing of years.

Nostalgia looses from memory the times and places of the soul, colors and shades of the past that have been obscured by oblivion and ripe for rediscovery, to be relived in all their luminous manifestations of meaning. It is true that nostalgia is premised upon the disposition to meditation and to internalization of the experiences that life puts us through, and expresses the desire not to let the past, its riches, its wounds die within us, but grants them a new life, an ebullient vital force that cannot but be open to the present and to the future. Nostalgia and its attendant concerns of the soul make our lives more sensitive to the lost values of youth that are within us, allowing us to grasp those things in others as well. And so, my discussion here has resonances I consider fostered by the values reflected in the vast territories of care that in psychiatry can never dispense with listening and dialogue.

The White Morning Stars

I don't know whether these pages of mine will be useful for sketching out the ongoing paths that guide us to the rediscovery of nostalgia, today so easily lost in the maelstrom of indifference and apathy, distraction and erasure of the past; regardless, my hope is that these pages have indicated the destinations to which nostalgia may lead in its path to understanding, which naturally will include interruptions and obstacles, but vertiginously broadens the borders of memory while reducing those of forgetting. The literary and philosophical excerpts, and especially the poetry, are, like the white stars of morning, linked to my personal and clinical experiences in endowing nostalgia with a maieutic function, helping nostalgia to be reborn from the past, from childhood and adolescence, forms of life that are reflected in the stages of adulthood, and developing it into hope, to take leaps, in ways that would be impossible any other way. In any case, whoever reads this book is called upon to answer my dauntless question as to whether it is possible to give life, to give meaning, to nostalgia wounded by carelessness and neglect, recovering its lost traces.

Blithe, Fair-Haired Inge

Now, in this last part of the present text, I would like to cite an excerpt from a tale of Thomas Mann's youth, *Tonio Kröger*, which is woven through with the sweet, aching nostalgia for a youth wounded by an unrequited love. Is this not often the reason for a nostalgia that follows us painfully through the course of our lives?

The protagonist of the story, the titular Tonio Kröger, at age sixteen falls in love with the blonde Inge, but this love is impossible: "That evening her image remained imprinted on his mind: her thick blond tresses, her rather narrowly cut laughing blue eyes, the delicate hint of freckles across the bridge of her nose. The timbre of her voice haunted him and he could not sleep; he tried softly to imitate the particular way she had pronounced that insignificant word, and a tremor ran through him as he did so. He knew from experience that this was love. And he knew only too well that love would cost him much pain, distress and humiliation; he knew also that it destroys the lover's peace of mind, flooding his heart with music and leaving him no time to form and shape his experience, to recollect it in tranquility and forge it into a whole. Nevertheless he accepted this love with joy, abandoning himself to it utterly and nourishing it with all the strength of his spirit." But this love is not mutual: "He loved Inge Holm, blithe, fair-haired Inge, who certainly despised him for his poetical scribblings... He watched her, he watched her narrow blue eyes so full of happiness and mockery; and an envious longing burned in his heart, a bitter insistent pain at the thought that to her he would always be an outsider and a stranger..."

His nostalgia for blithe, blonde, blue-eyed Inge would never wane, his heart would ache at the thought of her, and he would feel lost, ravaged, mortified, and ill, inconsolable with grief and nostalgia. But in a letter to a friend, and with this, the tale closes, Tonio Kröger writes, reconciled to his past: "Do not disparage this love, Lisaveta; it is good and fruitful. In it there is longing, and sad envy, and just a touch of contempt, and a whole world of innocent delight."

The nostalgia for lost love may burn so bright that it never flares out across the course of a lifetime, and Thomas Mann's story, immersed in the Heraclitean river of adolescent memory, is an unforgettable, sensuous testimony to its tenderness and delicacy, its magnanimity and melancholy, which brings me to conclude the present work on the nostalgia and its innumerable manifestations, its passions and metamorphoses.

Farewell

As I said at the beginning of these pages, phenomenology, even in psychiatry, is at bottom nothing more than a passion for difference, and following this epistemological path, I have tried to indicate the ways in which, the forms in which, nostalgia may be expressed, and which emotional and existential resonances it can take on within us as our lives unfold. It has, perhaps, not been a futile effort: at the least, it has allowed me to bring again to the surface for consideration, with the aid of psychiatry and literature, the multiple figures of nostalgia, which mediates our communication with the boundless worlds of interiority and memory. This work has been composed gradually, page by page, as happens, I would say, when a theme touches on an interest nourished on the arcane regions of the heart without which very little could be said about such human experiences as nostalgia, which is so fragile and at the bottom so ineffable, so shadowy and yet so like the stars.

This is how we live, and we are ever saying farewell to parts of ourselves which nostalgia later mysteriously allows us to rediscover.

Bibliography

Agamben, G., *Che cosa resta?* quodlibet.it. https://www.quodlibet.it/giorgio-agamben-che-cosa-resta. June 13, 2017.

Augustine, Saint. *The Confessions of St. Augustine*. Translated by Albert C. Outler.

Baldi, Guido, Silvia Giusto, and Giuseppe Zaccaria (eds). *Il piacere dei testi. Giacomo Leopardi*. Paravia: 2012.

Benjamin, Walter. *Selected Writings Volume 1: 1913-1926*. Michael W. Jennings, ed. Harvard University Press, 1996.

A Childhood in Berlin Around 1900. Translated by Howard Eiland. Belknap: 2006.

Bernanos, Georges. *The Carmelites*. Translated by Gerard Hopkins. Fontana: 1961.

Borgna, Eugenio. *L'arcipelago delle emozioni*. Feltrinelli: 2001.

L'ascolto gentile. Einaudi: 2017.

Celan, Paul. *Die Gedichte: Neue kommentierte Gesamtausgabe*, Suhrkamp: 2018.

Denisen, Isak. *Out of Africa*. Random House: 1992.

Dickinson, Emily. *The Letters of Emily Dickinson*. Belknap: 2024.

The Poems of Emily Dickinson. Variorum Edition. Belknap: 1998.

Dostoevsky, Fyodor. *The Brothers Karamazov*. Translated by David McDuff. Penguin Classics: 2003.

Freud, Sigmund. *The Standard Edition of the Complete Psychological Works of Sigmund Freud, vol. XIV*. Translated by James Strachey. The Hogarth Press: 1957.

Galimberti, Umberto. *Parole nomadi*. Feltrinelli: 1994.

Gozzano, Guido. *The Man I Pretend to Be*. Translated by Michael Palma. Princeton University Press: 1981.

Heidegger, Martin. *On the Way to Language*. HarperOne: 1982.

Hillesum, Etty. *An Interrupted Life: The Diaries and Letters from Westerbork 1941–1943*. Picador: 1996.

Hofmannsthal, Hugo von. *The Lyrical Poems of Hugo von Hofmannsthal.* Translated by Charles Wharton Stork. Yale University Press: 1918. *Buch der Freunde.* 1922.

Hölderlin, Friedrich. *Poems and Fragments.* Translated by Michael Hamburger. Anvil Press: 2004.

Leopardi, Giacomo. *Canti.* Translated by Jonathan Galassi. FSG: 2011.

Leopardi, Giacomo. *Zibaldone.* Translated by Michael Caesar et al. FSG: 2015.

Leopardi, Giacomo. *The Letters of Giacomo Leopardi 1817-1837.* Translated by Prue Shaw. Routledge: 1998.

Magris, Claudio. *L'anello di Clarisse.* Einaudi: 1984.

Mann, Thomas. *The Magic Mountain.* Translated by H.T. Lowe-Porter. Knopf: 1955. *Death in Venice and other Stories.* Translated by David Luke. Bantam Classics: 1988. *Essays of Three Decades.* Translated by H.T. Lowe-Porter. Knopf: 1947.

Milner, Max. *Georges Bernanos.* Desclée de Brouwer: 1967.

Mirabelli, Chiara. *Nostalgie. Sguardi sul dolore del ritorno.* Philo: 2012.

Musil, Robert. *The Confusions of Young Törless.* Continuum: 1986.

Nabokov, Vladimir. *Speak, Memory.* Vintage: 1989.

Nerval, Gérard de. *Selected Writings.* Penguin Classics, 1989.

Pascoli, Giovanni. "A Kite." Seamus Heaney, translator. In *Auguri: To Mary Kelleher*, edited by Maeve Binchy et al. Royal Dublin Society: 2009.

Petri, Rolf. "Nostalgia e Heimat. Emozione, tempo e spazinella costruzione dell'identità", in *Nostalgia. Memoria e passaggi tra le sponde dell'Adriatico.* Edizioni di Storia e Letteratura: 2010.

Potthoff, Elisabetta. "Vento antico," in Rainer Maria Rilke, *Vento e destino. Poesie, prose, sogni e appunti a Capri e a Napoli.* l'ancora del mediterraneo: 2006.

Proust, Marcel. *Swann's Way.* Translated by Lydia Davis. Penguin: 2002.

Rilke, Rainer Maria. *The Duino Elegies and the Sonnets to Orpheus.* Translated by A. Poulin, Jr. Houghton Mifflin: 1977.

The Notebooks of Malte Laurids Brigge. Translated by Michael Hulse. Penguin Classics: 2009.

Starobinski, Jean. *L'encre de la mélancholie*. Points: 2015.

Trakl, Georg. *Poems and Prose: A Bilingual Edition*. Translated by Alexander Stillmark. Northwestern University Press: 2005.

Ungaretti, Giuseppe. *Collected Poems, 1920-1954: Revised Bilingual Edition*. Translated by Jonathan Galassi. FSG: 2012.

Weil, Simone. *Waiting for God*. Translated by Emma Craufurd. Harper Colophon: 1973.

Weil, Simone. *Intimations of Christianity Among the Ancient Greeks*. Translated by Elisabeth Woolf, Virginia. *A Writer's Diary*. Houghton Mifflin: 2003.

Woolf, Virginia. *The Waves*. Penguin Classics: 2019.

Zambrano, María. *Algunos lugares de la poesía*. Trotta: 2007.

VECTORS

DEFINITION
Vectors are not like typical academic monographs. They are aimed at a more general audience, which might include undergraduate students, academics working in other fields, practitioners, policymakers, and the public. They provide a platform for established academic authors to reach a larger audience than usual, or to speak to new audiences; to deliver bold new arguments; to write unencumbered by the usual obligations for referencing; and to be exciting, provocative and even polemical.

ALREADY PUBLISHED:
Massimo Arcangeli, *Genderless Grammar.*
Alberto Lucarelli, *Tradition & Revolution.*
Eugenio Borgna, *Hope and Despair.*
Eugenio Borgna, *Wounded Nostalgia.*
Eugenio Borgna, *The Madness That is Also in Us.*

COMING SOON:
Simone Gozzano, *Consciousness.*

www.ingramcontent.com/pod-product-compliance
Lightning Source LLC
La Vergne TN
LVHW051607080426
835510LV00020B/3176